I0427388

Nature's Beauty

pure, natural, affordable

health and beauty solutions

ANGELA DE SOUZA

BISAC: HEA010000

Health & Fitness / Healthy Living

NATURE'S BEAUTY

CONTENTS

DISCLAIMER

This book is not intended as a substitute for the advice of medical doctors. The reader should regularly consult a medical doctor in matters relating to his/her health and particularly with respect to any symptoms that may require diagnosis or medical attention.

Nature's Beauty is my collection of alternatives to modern health and beauty products. I am not a doctor or a scientist, I don't have any letters after my name and am not trying to be someone I am not. I am offering some facts based on research, the findings from my own experiments and the findings from others who have joined me on this quest.

ANGELA DE SOUZA

INTRODUCTION

I am repeatedly outraged when I discover how many dangerous ingredients there are in what we put in and on our body. It has to stop, how will we live long and healthy lives if we are polluting our body with chemicals? Hi, I am Angela, wife and mother of four who loves her family very much and will do whatever I can to take care of them.

My passion, as you can tell, is my family, and this passion has led me to find ways to take care of them. Many years ago I discovered the importance of organic food, avoiding foods with 'E' numbers, hydrogenated vegetable oil, Aspartame and other such ingredients. More recently, I have discovered how harmful our shampoos, conditioners, toothpaste, air fresheners, washing up liquid and other such items, are.

Nature's Beauty is simply me sharing what I have found out with you. I am not a scientist but a mother. Where scientist's information has been used I will make sure I quote the source so you know clearly what you are reading. I hope you enjoy discovering all the fascinating things that I have discovered and most importantly, go on an adventure and discover even more yourself.

EWG

For more information visit the Environmental Working Group website www.ewg.org. At EWG, their team of scientists, engineers, policy experts, lawyers and computer programmers pore over government data, legal documents, scientific studies and have their own laboratory tests to expose threats to your health and the environment, and to find solutions. Their research brings to light unsettling facts that you have a right to know. All tables with data are from the EWG website.

DANGEROUS INGREDIENTS

Let's take a look at the top dangerous ingredients in most health and beauty products. Even if you decide not to use Nature's Way recipes for your health and beauty regime, do try and avoid products that contain these ingredients.

It is essential to understand that many ingredients in small quantities are harmless but consider how many of your products contain the same harmful ingredients. It is the cocktail of these ingredients that can kill us so don't be fooled when a company explains how a harmful ingredient in their particular product is below the harmful limit. It may well be, but how do you know how an ingredient in one product will react with another or how they compound in your body?

Do not believe that just because a product is labelled as 'natural' that it is free from these dangerous ingredients. Most common brands of 'natural' cleansers still use these harmful chemicals as their main active ingredient so it is essential to check your labels!

Sodium Lauryl Sulfate is probably the most dangerous ingredient used in skin, teeth and hair-care products. It is used in 90% of products that foam from things such as toothpaste to garage floor- cleaners and engine degreasers. It is a powerful and dangerous ingredient.

A report published in the Journal of The American College of Toxicology in 1983 showed that concentrations as low as 0.5% could cause irritation and concentrations of 10-30% caused skin corrosion and severe irritation. Consider that some soaps have concentrations of up to 30%.

Shampoos are among the most frequently reported products to the FDA. Reports include eye irritation, scalp irritation, tangled hair, swelling of the hands, face and arms as well as split and frizzy hair.

Perhaps most worryingly is that Sodium Lauryl Sulfate

is also absorbed into the body through the skin. Once it has been absorbed, one of the main effects is that it mimics the activity of Oestrogen. This has many health implications and is known to cause various premenstrual and menopausal symptoms as well as an increase in **female cancers** and decrease in male fertility.

Aspartame is one of the most dangerous substances on the market that is added to our foods. It is E951 - an artificial sweetener used in over 6000 products. Aspartame has been the subject of several controversies since its initial approval by the U.S. Food and Drug Administration (FDA) in 1974. In 2007, the UK supermarket chains Sainsbury's, M&S, and Asda, announced that they would no longer use aspartame in their own label products.

Aspartame accounts for over 75 percent of the adverse reactions to food additives reported to the FDA. Many of these reactions are very serious including seizures and death. A few of the 90 different documented symptoms listed in the report as being caused by aspartame include: Headaches/migraines, dizziness, seizures, nausea, numbness, muscle spasms, weight gain, rashes, depression, fatigue, irritability, tachycardia, insomnia, vision problems, hearing loss, heart palpitations, breathing difficulties, anxiety attacks, slurred speech, loss of taste, tinnitus, vertigo, memory loss, and joint pain.[i]

Flouride can be really dangerous if we have too much of it. Did you know that fluoride can damages sperm, damage bones and cause early puberty in children? *"It is apparent that fluorides have the ability to interfere with the functions of the brain."* — The National Research Council (2006). There are so many dangers, too many to list. The important thing to know is that fluoride is not only in toothpaste but also in our tap water so it is essential to filter drinking water as well as use toothpaste that is fluoride free. In some countries, fluoride is even added to table salt. A study published in the *Journal of the American Dental Association* confirmed fluoride as a toxic substance that actually destroys teeth, particularly those of developing young children and babies.

Fragrances which are found in most products are deceptively dangerous as fragrance on a label can indicate the presence of up to 4,000 separate ingredients, many toxic.

Parabens are found in almost all moisturisers and can cause irritation and allergic reactions. Reading University and Edinburgh Breast Unit Research Group found higher than average levels of parabens in breast tumour tissue.

Formaldehyde is a cheap preservative used in shampoo, conditioner, shower gel and childrens bubble bath. It has already been banned in Sweden and Japan as it is a cancer suspect and an irritant that can trigger allergies.

Nitrosamines are compounds which are used as wetting agents in facial cleansers, body washes and shampoos and are often present as contaminants. They have been shown to cause cancer in laboratory animals when taken orally.

There are many other dangerous products and it's best to do some research if you are concerned about a particular ingredient in your products.

ANGELA DE SOUZA

TEETH

Toothpaste

Toothpaste manufacturers would like us to believe that the only proper way to care for our teeth is with expensive, highly flavoured toothpastes that come in non-biodegradable tubes. What they don't tell you is that there are risks with using toothpaste, especially for children if they have fluoride.

Fluoride is poisonous! Although it could be helpful to our teeth in low dosage, chronic exposure to fluoride in large amounts interferes with bone formation. In this way, the greatest examples of fluoride poisoning arise from fluoride-rich ground water. In advanced countries, most cases of fluoride exposure are due to the ingestion of dental fluoride products.

Although exposure to these products does not often cause toxicity, in one study thirty percent of children exposed to fluoride dental products developed mild symptoms[ii].

Symptoms of fluoride poisoning can include abdominal pain, diarrhoea, hyper salivation, nausea and vomiting. Neurological symptoms include headaches, muscle weakness, hyperactive reflexes and muscular spasms. In severe cases, multi-organ failure will occur.

Children can also experience gastrointestinal distress upon ingesting sufficient amounts of flavoured toothpaste. Adults and children alike are also exposed to harmful, artificial sweeteners in toothpaste which are toxic to your body.[iii]

The following table shows the health concerns based on commonly used whitening toothpaste.

Health concerns of ingredients

	low ▼	moderate ▼	high ▼
Overall Hazard	▓▓▓▓▓▓		
Cancer	▓		
Developmental & reproductive toxicity	▓▓▓▓		
Allergies & immunotoxicity	▓▓▓		
Use restrictions	▓▓▓▓		

Other HIGH concerns: Neurotoxicity, Persistence and bioaccumulation, Organ system toxicity (non-reproductive), Miscellaneous, Multiple, additive exposure sources, Irritation (skin, eyes, or lungs)

Other LOW concerns: Ecotoxicology, Data gaps, Enhanced skin absorption, Contamination concerns, Occupational hazards

Nature's Way Alternatives

Dental care is so simple in many ways. Our body is designed to heal itself, so if we are consistent with preventative methods then our body should take care of the rest. My solution is simple - Bicarbonate of Soda. By sprinkling a little dry powder on a dry toothbrush and brushing, you have your toothpaste problems solved. It's safe for adults and children.

Bicarbonate of Soda is a soft, dissolvable, mild abrasive substance that kills bacteria and all of the microorganisms associated with infections. It will also prevent plaque build up by neutralizing and detoxifying bacterial acids and toxins.

Results:

- Clean teeth
- Fresh breath
- Kills germs and bacteria
- Nicer 'morning' breath
- Save money

Cautions:

- Inflamed and bleeding gums

Eric used Bicarbonate of Soda twice a day but his gums became inflamed and had some slight bleeding. We discovered that this was due to the fact that he brushed his teeth in an up and down motion rather than in small circles. Also he brushed his teeth with a hard toothbrush and applied a lot of pressure when brushing. After brushing less harshly and in a circular motion, his gums returned to normal. I have also read though, that it is common to have some bleeding after a deep clean, even at the dentist, as the tartar build up from around the gums is removed causing some bleeding.

NATURE'S WAY TOOTHPASTE

Ingredients: Bicarbonate of Soda

Method: Sprinkle Bicarbonate of Soda onto your toothbrush and brush your teeth in small circles. Lightly brush your tongue too.

For added benefits put a couple of drops of diluted distilled vinegar or apple cider vinegar on your toothbrush*.

---

*Vinegar helps to kill bacteria and prevent the build-up of calculus, more commonly known as tartar. Either brushing or rinsing with vinegar reduces the risk of gingivitis but always dilute the vinegar with plenty of water or it will be too strong and eat away at the enamel on your teeth.

More toothpastes recipes:

There are many recipes available for more complex toothpastes using natural ingredients, here are some examples:

Vinegar and Bicarbonate of Soda Toothpaste

- Mix 4 tbsp. Bicarbonate of Soda and glycerine into a paste.
- Add 5 drops of tea tree essential oil and 10 drops of peppermint essential oil.
- Use paste along with a drop of vinegar on top and brush.

Salt and Bicarbonate of Soda Toothpaste

- Grind 1 tbsp dried lemon or orange peel into a fine powder
- Mix powder into a paste with 1 tsp. Bicarbonate of Soda, 1 tsp. fine sea salt

Citrus Toothpaste

- Mix 6 tsp. Bicarbonate of Soda, ½ tsp. fine sea salt and 1 drop peppermint essential oil into a paste.

Try experimenting with your own toothpaste recipes.

My Toothpaste Experiment

Date Started_____   Date Ended_____

Recipe Used

_____

_____

_____

_____

_____

_____

Findings

_____

_____

_____

_____

_____

_____

Six month review

_____

_____

Melbourne University conducted a study of more than 3,200 people, which found a nine-fold increase in the risk of cancer among smokers and a five-fold rise among drinkers. The ethanol in mouthwash is thought to **help** cancer-causing substances – such as nicotine – permeate the mouth lining.[iv]

Nature's Way Alternatives

Mouthwash is simply for flushing your mouth to remove waste that is trapped. If your teeth and tongue are brushed correctly you don't need anything as harsh as alcohol to rinse your mouth. Something as simple as warm salt water will do the job just fine and from there the body's normal reparative process will take over. Our bodies naturally repair our gums and bones, the harsh products that we often use hinder this natural process. The best thing we can do is not get in the way and keep our dental hygiene routine as simple as possible.

Vinegar is another powerful plaque destroying mouthwash and can be used in the same way as salt, diluted in a cup of water.

If you would like a bit of taste or minty fragrance, add a couple of drops of peppermint essential oil with the salt or vinegar water.

Results:

- Enhanced oral hygiene
- Kills germs and bacteria
- Fresh breath
- Treatment for mouth infections and ulcers
- Save money

Take care when using vinegar though, it should be diluted with plenty of water as the acid can damage the enamel on your teeth if the concentration is too strong. After using a vinegar mouthwash or toothpaste, rinse well with water to flush away any remaining acid.

NATURE'S WAY MOUTHWASH

Ingredients: Vinegar or salt

Method: Dilute 1 teaspoon of vinegar or salt in a glass of warm water and use daily as a mouthwash. For added freshness, add a couple of drops of peppermint essential oil to your vinegar or salt water.

More mouthwash recipes:

There are many recipes available for more complex mouthwashes using natural ingredients, here are some examples:

Rosemary-Mint Mouthwash

- Add 1 tsp. of fresh mint leaves, 1 tsp of rosemary leaves and 1 tsp of anise seeds to 1 cup of water.
- Bring the water to boil and leave to infuse for 20 minutes.
- Remove from heat to cool, remove leaves and seeds to use as mouthwash.

Cardamom and Clove Mouthwash

- Add 1 tsp. of whole cloves and a pinch of ground cardamom to 1 cup of boiling water.
- Leave to cool and then strain out cloves and cardamom to use as mouthwash.

Cranberry Mouthwash

- Rinse your mouth with natural, unsweetened cranberry juice. You can also brush your teeth with cranberry juice and you can even swallow it afterwards if you want to!

My Mouthwash Experiment

Date Started_____   Date Ended_____

Recipe Used

_____

_____

_____

_____

_____

_____

Findings

_____

_____

_____

_____

_____

_____

Six month review

_____

_____

Whitening

Let's begin will dispelling the fallacy that teeth are pure white. Pure white teeth are not natural and the best way to tell what colour your teeth should be is to look at a child's teeth. If they are eating correctly then their tooth colour is the perfectly natural colour that our teeth should be. A tooth has a similar makeup to ivory and as you know ivory is not pure white either. The following table shows the health concerns based on common whitening products.

Health concerns of ingredients

	low ▼	moderate ▼	high ▼
Overall Hazard	███████████████		
Cancer	█████		
Developmental & reproductive toxicity	████████		
Allergies & immunotoxicity	████████████		
Use restrictions	██████████		

Other HIGH concerns: Neurotoxicity, Persistence and bioaccumulation, Organ system toxicity (non-reproductive), Miscellaneous, Multiple, additive exposure sources, Irritation (skin, eyes, or lungs), Contamination concerns, Occupational hazards

Other LOW concerns: Endocrine disruption, Ecotoxicology, Data gaps

Stained or yellow teeth can be caused by what we eat and drink, as well as poor dental hygiene. Removing stains as opposed to whitening through bleaching is best for your teeth. Bleaching your teeth might give you sparkling white teeth for a few months or years but could cause you a life time of teeth problems afterwards. Keep your teeth clean and remove stains but don't go for the pure white, unnatural look as that is a sure sign that problems will follow later on in life.

Nature's Way Alternatives

1. Eat Your Teeth Clean

The most natural way to keep your teeth free from stains is to eat vegetables such as celery, carrots, broccoli and cucumbers. These vegetables are naturally abrasive and have the same effect as brushing and whitening your teeth without any harmful consequences.

2. Brush with Bicarbonate of Soda

This remains the most effective, safe and natural whitening method. Many harmful whitening toothpastes contain Bicarbonate of Soda as their main whitening ingredient. Why not skip all the added dangerous ingredients and only use Bicarbonate of Soda?

3.   Clean with a Microfiber Cloth

Try rubbing your teeth with a microfiber cloth when your teeth start looking a little dull. You might just see the dirt rub off onto the cloth which means the discolouration was merely stains from coffee, tea or wine.

4.   Rinse after Drinking

A fantastic way to avoid staining is to rinse your mouth with water immediately after drinking tea, coffee, cola or wine. Of course brushing is best but simply rinsing will remove most of the tea, coffee, cola or wine that is known to stain teeth.

Results:
- Whiter, cleaner teeth
- Enhanced oral hygiene
- Save money

Cautions:
- Avoid using fruit such as lemons and strawberries regularly for whitening. If you want the natural whitening effect of lemons and strawberries just eat them normally, don't rub them onto your teeth or leave their juice on your teeth for a long period of time. Although you will see instant whitening

results, the acid will strip away the tooth enamel until it is damaged beyond repair. If you choose to use fruit for whitening, brush your teeth afterwards and rinse your mouth well.

- Some people use Peroxide as a whitener. This is a common ingredient in tooth whiteners and it will whiten your teeth but bleaching molecules can get trapped in nerve passageways which can cause increased tooth sensitivity. If you choose to use peroxide don't leave it on your teeth for too long.

NATURE'S WAY WHITENING

Ingredients: Celery, carrots, broccoli and cucumbers

Method: Eat one or more of these vegetables every day and enjoy perfect colour teeth. For added whiteness continue brushing with Bicarbonate of Soda.

My Teeth Whitening Experiment

Date Started_____   Date Ended_____

Recipe Used

_____

_____

_____

_____

_____

_____

Findings

_____

_____

_____

_____

_____

_____

Six month review

_____

_____

Food for Teeth

Celery

Celery is made up of 90% water. Eating celery inhibits bacterial growth and it helps you with the general cleaning of teeth. Celery also massages gums and cleans between the teeth.

Onion

Onion contains antibacterial elements which are powerful in the prevention of tooth decay. Fresh onion is best.

Milk, Yoghurt and Cheese

These foods contain calcium which is essential for strong bones and teeth. Unsweetened milk and yoghurt have a low acidity which reduces dental erosion. Cheese helps balance your mouth's pH and rebuilds tooth enamel.

Sesame Seeds

Sesame seeds are high in calcium and helps build tooth enamel and prevent plaque build up.

Strawberries and Citrus

Eating strawberries and other fruit high in vitamin C also strengthens your teeth and gums.

Did you know?

- The alcohol in commercially produced mouthwash can cause permanent bad breath.
- Sugarless gum isn't good for your teeth. Check out the ingredients list on your gum and you will see that a large percentage is carbohydrates, which can be just as bad as sugar. The bacteria that cause tooth decay will survive and breed on those carbohydrates.

Fresh Breath Tips:

1. If you want to add some flavour to your 'bicarb toothpaste' mix in some cinnamon.
2. Chew on a fresh leave of mint, it does wonders for your breath, or chew on dried coriander leaves.
3. Gargle with one teaspoon of ginger juice and one teaspoon of lemon juice in a glassful of warm water.

HAIR

Shampoo

I was shocked when I discovered that the dangerous chemicals in shampoos were found not only in your every day cheap shampoos but also in luxury salon shampoos, shampoos claiming to be natural or organic and even baby shampoos. In fact, some of my research led to me to a shocking discovery about a very popular brand of baby shampoo. This shampoo contained three carcinogenic ingredients namely dioxane, formaldehyde and nitrosamine.

It's terribly complicated with many scientific explanations which I will not be going into but the bottom line is that these ingredients are extremely dangerous. Scientific information on all of the ingredients listed on your shampoo bottles can be easily obtained on the internet. Here is a list of some of the dangerous ingredients to look out for:

- Quaternium-15
- DMDM hydantoin
- Imidazolidinyl urea
- Diazolidinyl urea
- PEG-100 stearate
- Sodium laureth sulfate
- Sodium myreth sulfate
- Polyethylene
- Ceteareth-20
- Propylene Glycol
- Methyl paraben, ethyl paraben, propyl paraben, butyl paraben, isobutyl paraben or E216

The 2007 EWG study[v] also determined that:

- *82 percent of children are exposed every week to one or more ingredients with the potential to harm the brain and nervous system.*

- *69 percent of children are exposed every week to one or more ingredients that may disrupt the hormone system.*

- *3.6 percent of children are exposed to ingredients with strong data linking them to cancer, including chemicals classified as known or probable human carcinogens.*

- *80 percent of children's products marked as gentle and non-irritating contain ingredients linked to allergies and skin or eye irritation according to government and industry sources.*

The bottom line, however, is that if you are not sure what the ingredients on the shampoo bottle label mean then perhaps stay away from it. If you can't pronounce it, you probably don't want to put it on your body anyway. Each country will offer different ingredients in their shampoos as each country has different regulations.

Nature's Way Alternatives

Shampoo does not have to lather and does not need to be complicated. More often than not we suffer from dry hair, itchy scalp, oily hair or other common problems as a **result** of all the shampoo we use! Your body produces oil to keep your hair naturally healthy. Using shampoo upsets this natural balance and could cause you to produce more oil than is necessary. Shampoo also irritates your scalp and hair which could cause it to dry out. The simplest 'shampoo' is one tablespoon of Bicarbonate of Soda mixed with two tablespoons of water. It works by opening up the scales of the hair shaft then combining with our natural oils to clean our hair. At first it might feel strange as there is no lather and you really need to work it through your hair well while being gentle on your scalp. Allow two to four weeks for your hair to adjust. Your hair may become dry, frizzy or oily as it adjusts but eventually everything will level out and you will reap the benefits and have fantastic hair.

Results:
- No harmful chemicals
- Clean hair
- Balanced natural oils
- Save money

Cautions:
- Bicarbonate of soda might strip the colour from some coloured hair.
- Bicarbonate of Soda is known to have a slight lightening effect on some hair types.
- Bicarbonate of soda can dry hair if used too often.

I have been using Bicarbonate of Soda to wash my hair once or twice a week for six months and will never go back to using shampoo. I also use this method on my children, aged three and six years old, and have not only found their hair to be shinier and healthier but have also noticed that their eczema has totally cleared up.

NATURE'S WAY SHAMPOO

Ingredients: Bicarbonate of Soda

Method: Mix one tablespoon of Bicarbonate of Soda with two tablespoons of water. Work the paste through your hair and rinse thoroughly.

More shampoo recipes:

Olive Oil and Grapeseed Shampoo

- 1/4 cup water
- 1/4 cup liquid Castile Soap (Olive Oil soap)
- 1 teaspoon grapeseed oil
- Mix ingredients together, wash and rinse well.

Honey and Mustard Shampoo

- ½ teaspoon probiotic yoghurt
- 1 teaspoon mustard powder
- 1 teaspoon honey
- 1 teaspoon grapeseed oil

Dilute 1 teaspoon of mustard powder with yoghurt and then add honey and grapeseed oil. Apply the mixture on your hair and massage into your scalp then rinse. For extra conditioning leave in for 20 minutes and then rinse very well with water.

To get rid of excess oils you might like to do a mild Bicarbonate of Soda wash afterwards.

My Hair Shampoo Experiment

Date Started_____   Date Ended_____

Recipe Used

_____

_____

_____

_____

_____

_____

Findings

_____

_____

_____

_____

_____

_____

Six month review

_____

_____

Conditioner

Out of all my research, conditioner has turned up as one of the most harmful of all the products we have looked at thus far. Even the children's conditioners and some of the organic ones have shown cancer risks.

Marianne Kapfer, a librarian in Washington, D.C., likes a natural look. She doesn't wear much makeup but loves to indulge in a good shampoo and conditioner. When she started reading labels more closely, however, "I realized that my 'natural' shampoo wasn't so natural," Marianne says. And that's not all. Due to labelling loopholes, many 'natural' and 'organic' personal-care products in the United States contain hazardous chemicals, some of which, at high exposures, have been shown to cause cancer, birth defects, damage to nervous and reproductive systems and liver damage in lab animals.[vi]

Sadly, you cannot assume that a conditioner that says it's 'natural' or 'organic' is safe. You either need to know your ingredients really well and scrutinise the labels or simply stick to ingredients from your fruit bowl or refrigerator. A great guideline is - if you won't eat it, don't put it on your body. Your skin absorbs everything so there is little difference between what you put into your body and what you put onto your body. Either way it is absorbed into your blood stream and distributed throughout your body.

The following table shows the health concerns based on commonly used conditioner.

Health concerns of ingredients

	low	moderate	high
Overall Hazard	▓▓▓▓▓▓▓▓▓▓▓▓▓▓		
Cancer	▓▓▓▓▓		
Developmental & reproductive toxicity	▓▓▓▓▓▓▓▓▓▓▓▓▓▓▓▓▓		
Allergies & immunotoxicity	▓▓▓▓▓▓▓▓▓▓		
Use restrictions	▓▓▓▓▓▓▓▓▓▓		

Other HIGH concerns: Miscellaneous, Multiple, additive exposure sources, Irritation (skin, eyes, or lungs), Contamination concerns, Occupational hazards, Biochemical or cellular level changes

Other MODERATE concerns: Neurotoxicity, Organ system toxicity (non-reproductive)

Nature's Way Alternatives

Vinegar is the best conditioner and hair detangler. I have tried all sorts of natural conditioners but keep coming back to plain and simple white distilled vinegar. It's cheap and works amazingly well on the whole family. The only thing I would say is that it does burn your eyes or open wounds. Take special care when using it on children as you don't want to burn their eyes. The results are fantastic though, it cures dandruff and an itchy scalp and leaves you with a brilliant, natural shine.

Another great alternative to vinegar is lemon juice. This has a similar effect to vinegar without the vinegar smell. These acids strengthen the hydrogen bonds in hair protein and help seal the outer layer of the cuticle. Lemon juice however, will lighten your hair over a long period of time whereas vinegar will not have the same effect. Lemon juice is also great for washing your face, so you can allow it to run onto your face and do two things at once, but we will get to that in the next chapter.

Results:

- No dandruff or itchy scalp
- Save money
- Great shine
- No tangles
- No harmful chemicals

Cautions:

- Avoid contact with eyes

- Will sting open wounds but is not harmful to them
- Rinse vinegar well or you will smell like a fish and chips shop!

NATURE'S WAY CONDITIONER

Ingredients: Vinegar

Method: Pour undiluted distilled white vinegar into your hair. Massage gently into your scalp and rinse well.

More conditioner recipes:

There are many recipes available for conditioners using natural ingredients, here are some examples:

Guar Gum Conditioner

- 1 cup water
- ⅛ teaspoon Guar Gum*[1]
- 1 teaspoon grapeseed oil

---

[1] Guar Gum is available on eBay or Amazon and in some supermarkets.

Mix the Guar Gum into a paste by slowly adding small amounts of water. Once all the gum is mixed together slowly add the rest of the water. Next add the oil and either whisk or shake the container until the oil is mixed well. Store this conditioner in the fridge for use up one month. Use as conditioner and either rinse out or leave in.

Aloe Vera and Lemon Conditioner

- ¼ cup Aloe Vera gel
- Juice from ½ lemon

Apply to washed hair, leave it in for five minutes and then rinse.

Alternatively, rub a small amount of Aloe Vera gel into your hair as a leave in conditioner.

Honey Conditioner

- Mix equal parts of honey and water.

Work the mixture through your hair and then rinse with warm water. Several rinses may be necessary to remove the honey but the result will be incredible soft and silky hair. Manuka honey is best and it has been said that it can even help with hair loss problems by rejuvenating the scalp and encouraging hair growth over time.

Beer Conditioner

- 1 cup flat beer

After shampooing, pour the beer through your hair and let it sit for a few minutes. Massage your scalp gently and make sure the beer touches the roots of your hair. Rinse very well or your hair will smell like beer. The proteins and sugars in the beer will strengthen the Keratin in your hair and give it a fantastic shine. To get rid of the shine you could give your hair a rinse with an essential oil or boil some mint in some water and when it has cooled, rinse your hair with the minty water.

Coconut Milk Leave in Conditioner

- Coconut Milk

Towel dry your hair.

Before applying the coconut milk, shake the coconut milk container very well as it usually comes separated.

Pour a little coconut milk into your palms and work it through your hair starting about an inch away from your roots.

Be careful not to use too much as your hair will go very greasy.

Personally, for my hair type I found the leave in conditioner option too greasy but it worked fantastic once I rinsed the coconut milk out. It's best to experiment as everyone has different hair. If you do happen to end up with your hair too greasy, there is no need to wash it again. Simply give your hair a good rinse with vinegar which will break down some of the oiliness from the coconut milk but not totally remove it. The results are fantastic. Be sure to rinse the vinegar out well though so you don't lose too much of the coconut fragrance and replace it with the smell of vinegar.

My Hair Conditioner Experiment

Date Started_____   Date Ended_____

Recipe Used

_____

_____

_____

_____

_____

_____

Findings

_____

_____

_____

_____

_____

_____

Six month review

_____

_____

Serum & Heat Protector

As with all hair care products, serums and heat protectors can come with high health risks and may contain several cancer causing ingredients. Most of these products contain silicones such as Cyclomethicone and Dimethicone. These silicones are heavy and very difficult to wash out and more importantly may interfere with hormone function and damage the liver. Logically, if you think about it, silicone coats the hair, trapping anything beneath it, and does not allow the hair to breathe. Silicones do give the hair a shine at first by coating the hair strands with oils but these oils are extremely bad for the hair. Long term use will only make your hair worse, not better.

Nature's Way Alternatives

Natural oils help to enhance absorbability of other natural ingredients to promote healing of damaged hair shaft. These oils are fantastic both as serum and as a heat protector. I have found that extra virgin Olive Oil Oil and grapeseed oil are fantastic oils for these and many other purposes.

Grapeseed oil is a great heat protector as it has a very high smoke point. Olive Oil also has a high smoke point but not as high as grapeseed oil. The smoke point generally refers to the temperature at which the oil begins to break down to glycerol and free fatty acids which produce bluish smoke. When using natural oil make sure that you are not heating it to the smoke point.

Grapeseed oil is a light, gentle oil that is high in linoleic acid and vitamin E. Vitamin E is vital in hair and skin care as it is one of the most powerful natural antioxidants which helps to combat free radicals and other damaging elements in the skin. These factors make grapeseed oil an excellent oil not only for moisturising your hair, but also in protecting your hair from hair damaging hair dryers, hot irons, etc.

Personally, I have found Olive Oil fantastic for my hair since my hair is very fine and often frizzy. The Olive Oil holds my hair down well avoiding the flyaway look and at the same time giving it a fantastic shine. Remember to use it sparingly to avoid your hair getting overly greasy.

Results:
- Save money
- Healthier hair
- Natural shine
- Nourishment rather than coating
- Heat protection

Cautions:

- Too much oil looks terrible on hair. Start with applying very little oil and slowly add more if required.
- Be careful to apply the oil evenly or you may not notice that the back of your hair is greasy while the front looks great!

NATURE'S WAY SERUM & HEAT PROTECTOR

Ingredients: Extra Virgin Olive Oil or Grapeseed Oil

Method: For use as serum or heat protector, take the bottle of oil and hold it tightly against the palm of your hand. Turn the bottle upside down onto your hand for a second or two which will leave you with a small amount of oil in your palm. Two or three drops of oil this size is all you need (depending on the length of your hair). Rub the oil between your palms and work it into your hair evenly by taking some hair into your hand from about an inch away from the roots and then sliding your hands lightly through your hair.

My Hair Serum & Heat Protector Experiment

Date Started_____   Date Ended_____

Recipe Used

_____

_____

_____

_____

_____

_____

Findings

_____

_____

_____

_____

_____

_____

Six month review

_____

_____

Hair Treatments

I struggled to find much information on hair treatments. It seems that the information is similar to that of a conditioner. If you know your ingredients and know what to avoid, you should be safe. Most hair treatments have a similar cancer risk to conditioners and shampoos. One thing stood out though and that was the new research on Keratin based treatments. Keratin is the latest thing to get frizz free hair. It is found in our body naturally and is a family of fibrous structural proteins that make up the outer layer of human skin and is also the key structural component of our hair and nails. When the Keratin in our body is damaged it makes our hair and skin look dull which is why many people tend to have a Keratin treatment.

These treatments are made by taking the Keratin from animals, like the wool from sheep, and making a mixture out of it. This mixture will be applied to the hair as a Keratin treatment to replenish the hair's damaged Keratin.

Sadly this seemingly 'natural' treatment is not natural at all and several side effects such as excessive hair loss, deterioration of hair condition, allergic reactions, and in some cases, cancer, has even been reported. As with all of these dangerous products, you hair will look great at first but after some time has passed you will begin to see the negative side effects.

The Brazilian Blowout is another popular hair treatment at the moment but sadly reports of similar bad side effects have started coming in recently. Most Keratin hair treatments use formaldehyde, which is a known carcinogen.

Why not stick to nature's way? Rather than try the latest new product that has not been thoroughly tested, use something that has been around since the beginning of time, something like Olive Oil or yoghurt.

Nature's Way Alternatives

Olive Oil is the best treatment for hair. Olive Oil nourishes and conditions your hair. It also improves the strength and elasticity of your hair. Unlike harmful chemical treatment, Olive Oil doesn't just coat your hair but it actually feeds it.

Olive Oil contains a wide variety of valuable antioxidants that are not found in other oils. In fact Olive Oil is known to protect us from certain types of cancer. It is also immensely beneficial in adding smoothness and softness to a dry scalp, especially during the winter months. All in all you cannot go wrong with Olive Oil.

Results:

- Healthy, shiny hair
- More manageable hair
- Save money
- Softer hair
- No harmful chemicals

Cautions:

- Take care to wash well or greasy hair will result.

NATURE'S WAY HAIR TREATMENT

Ingredients: Olive Oil

Method: Rinse your hair with warm water before washing. Warm one tablespoon of Olive Oil by rubbing it in the palms of your hands then gently massage the oil into your scalp.

Make sure that you rub plenty of oil on the ends of your hair. Place a plastic bag over your hair for half an hour.

Rinse extremely well with warm water and then shampoo as usual.

* You can also add fresh rosemary to the oil as rosemary is well known for its tonic effects and natural hair conditioning. Add a fresh sprig of rosemary to your bottle of oil and leave it there – it will add flavour to your cooking and will condition your hair.

More treatment recipes:

There are many other simple ways to give your hair a deep treatment using natural ingredients, here are some examples:

Yoghurt

Yoghurt has natural antifungal and antibacterial properties as well as many healthy enzymes along with natural oils. Using yoghurt in your hair stimulates hair growth and will also fight dandruff. The protein in yoghurt helps to strengthen and moisturise your hair.

Yoghurt Treatment

- ½ cup plain probiotic yoghurt

Mix the yoghurt well with a fork or put it in a blender for a couple of minutes. Part your hair and apply the yoghurt to your scalp until your entire scalp is covered with yoghurt. Then work the yoghurt through your hair with your fingers or with a wide toothed comb. Leave to soak for one hour and then rinse out well with warm water and wash as usual.

For extra strength and shine, beat an egg into the yoghurt and apply as above. Take care to rinse the yoghurt and egg treatment out with cool water as the egg will cook into your hair if you use warm water! I have found that the yoghurt can leave a terrible smell in your hair. Make sure you rinse very well and perhaps use an essential oil when washing your hair afterwards.

Hot Oil Treatment

- ½ cup of rosemary
- ½ cup Olive Oil

Mix oil and rosemary over low heat, stirring constantly until warm. Remove from heat and strain leaves from the oil. Work the warmed oil into your scalp to the ends of hair and then wrap your hair up in a plastic bag. Leave for 15 minutes then wash well.

Your Hair Treatment Experiment

Date Started_____   Date Ended_____

Recipe Used

_____

_____

_____

_____

_____

_____

Findings

_____

_____

_____

_____

_____

Six month review

_____

_____

Hair Colouring

Good news for those of you living in the EU but sadly bad news for my USA friends. Europe is well ahead of the USA in its responses to potentially dangerous chemicals in health and beauty products. On 1st December 2007 a ban was imposed on 22 hair dye substances issued by the European Commission. These ingredients had been linked to bladder cancer in a 2001 University of Southern California study. Günter Verheugen, the European Commission Vice-President, said, "*Substances for which there is no proof that they are safe will disappear from the market. Our high safety standards do not only protect EU consumers, they also give legal certainty to the European cosmetics industry.*" The USA however, has not required manufacturers to file data on ingredients or report cosmetic-related injuries. If you wish to find the exact 22 ingredients do an Internet search for '*Europe Bans 22 Hair Dye Chemicals*'

The most dangerous hair dye ingredients are the Arylamines chemicals. One of these is called Phenylenediamine (PPD) and is present in about seventy five percent of chemical hair dyes including non-permanent 'natural' products. It is known to be toxic to the immune system, skin, nervous system, respiratory system, liver and kidneys.

Despite the fact that many hair dyes are extremely

toxic many companies get away with using them by providing a warning on the box. Their warning states that you should not allow their hair dye to come into contact with the skin and because of this warning they can justify using the chemicals that they do. Sadly, as you may already know, you cannot avoid all contact with your skin. It either gets onto your hands somehow or most certainly touches your scalp in places. Once it has contact with the skin it is absorbed into your blood stream and released into your body. Laboratory experiments have shown that PPD damages the DNA of human cells and of course accumulated DNA damage leads to cancer.

These harmful chemicals are not only found in home hair dye kits but can also be found in salon dyes. It's essential to talk to your hair dresser and find out what ingredients are in the products they use. Many have died from ignorance. That is extreme but true. Even if you don't get cancer, you still risk losing your hair as many people have reported hair thinning and hair loss as a result of the chemicals in hair dyes.

The following table shows the health concerns based on commonly used hair dye.

Health concerns of ingredients

	low	moderate	high
	▼	▼	▼
Overall Hazard			
Cancer			
Developmental & reproductive toxicity			
Allergies & immunotoxicity			
Use restrictions			

Other HIGH concerns: Neurotoxicity, Endocrine disruption, Persistence and bioaccumulation, Organ system toxicity (non-reproductive), Miscellaneous, Multiple, additive exposure sources, Irritation (skin, eyes, or lungs), Contamination concerns, Occupational hazards

Other LOW concerns: Ecotoxicology, Data gaps, Enhanced skin absorption

Nature's Way Alternatives

Dark Hair

Henna is the best way to colour darker hair. Henna has been used for thousands of years and traces have even been found on the hair and beards of ancient Egyptian mummies. Henna acts like a hair varnish that coats the outside of your hair, protecting and coating the cuticle. The results are natural colours and a stunning shine. Either buy Henna in its pure leaf form or get a Henna block which also contains cocoa butter from *Lush*. The thing I like most about Henna is that it works with the natural colour of each strand of your hair. This means that you don't get only one shade in your hair which tends to look very unnatural but a gorgeous natural looking head of hair.

Results:

- Conditioned hair
- Natural shine
- Damage protection
- Stronger hair
- Reduction of dandruff
- No harmful chemicals

Cautions:

- In rare cases Henna has been known to turn hair green but there is a simple remedy – Henna over the top to build up a rich, not green, colour.
- Ensure you buy 100% natural Henna and not Henna with additives and this would completely

defeat the purpose of using Henna in the first place.

- Do a strand test first by colouring only a few strands to see if you get the desired result.

NATURE'S WAY DARK HAIR COLOUR

Ingredients: Henna

Method: Mix powder with water into a paste and apply to clean dry hair.

Protect your forehead from staining by rubbing some oil into your hairline before applying the Henna. Separate your hair into small sections and apply Henna from root to tip.

Cover your hair for a more red shade and leave uncovered for a brown tone. Leave in for minimum one hour, for best results leave in for four hours. Rinse really well and then wash as usual.

Usually detailed instructions accompany the Henna powder or the Henna blocks from *Lush*.

Light Hair:

Sunshine and lemon juice are the best ways to lighten hair. Lemon juice contains high concentrations of nourishing elements like vitamin C, vitamin B, and phosphorous, along with antioxidant properties. A sensible amount of sun is also very good for you as the sun produces Vitamin D in your body.

NATURE'S WAY LIGHT HAIR COLOUR

Ingredients: Lemon juice and Sun

Method: To use lemon juice and the sun, mix the juice of 1 fresh lemon with 8 tablespoons of water and rub it in to your dry hair. Leave in your hair for four hours and then rinse.

To speed up the process, lie in the sun. Cover your body with cloth (to avoid damage to your skin) and spread your hair out to absorb the rays.

Your Hair Colour Experiment

Date Started_____   Date Ended_____

Recipe Used

_____

_____

_____

_____

_____

_____

Findings

_____

_____

_____

_____

_____

_____

Six month review

_____

_____

Head Lice

This is not a nice subject but an important one to discuss, especially if you have young school age children. I wasn't sure whether or not to include this section as it's not very pleasant to talk about. However, I remember struggling with lice in my children's hair for about a year and it drove us crazy. At first we tried all the popular lice treatments but after a few months it seemed that the lice seemed immune to them. It was then that I beguan to research natural remedies and I did so mostly because of the high cost of the conventional methods. We did have success and managed to keep the lice at bay only to discover that as soon as my daughter left the school she was in, the lice problem stopped. Our problem was not lice treatment as much as it was another child in the school whose parents didn't bother with any lice treatment at all. So if you are having a long term lice problem, you might want to look into who the carrier is and have a nice little talk with them!

Sadly, most of the chemical-based head lice treatments contain pyrethrins and pesticides suspected of causing neurological damage. Children in particular have less well-developed immune systems and a number of studies have indicated that they have a higher sensitivity to pesticide toxins. Symptoms can include irritation, headaches, dizziness, acute hallucinations, hyperactivity, and a general lack of energy.

A London Times article of October 5, 1997 reported, "Alison and Keith Thomson from Carlisle started treating their three boys with the delousing lotion Derbac-M after an outbreak of nits at their local primary school last year. 'We kept treating them for about three or four months because they kept getting re-infected,' said Allison. 'I asked the doctor if it was okay to keep using it, and he said it was fine.' Just before Christmas Paul, 6, developed flu-like symptoms. He became lethargic and his personality changed. By Christmas he had become incontinent and could hardly walk. Doctors have said a possible cause is organophoaphates poisoning."

In that same article, Dr. Vyvyan Howard, senior lecturer in fetal and infant toxio-pathology at the University of Liverpool verified that possibility and added, "I have used these lotions [head lice treatments containing pesticides] myself in the past but knowing what I do now, I would never dream of using them again on my children."[vii]

It has also been reported that head lice are becoming resistant to common drug treatments. Overuse of pesticide treatments are endangering children; international media and medical literature are reporting that head lice are winning the war. These new "super lice" are becoming more and more resistant to the chemical based treatments. As a result, there is no chemical based lice treatment that is 100% effective against head lice.

Nature's Way Alternatives

Using natural shampoo and conditioners will automatically reduce your susceptibility to head lice. Using the Bicarbonate of Soda washing method and vinegar as a rinse makes your hair very slippery which means that the lice eggs cannot attach themselves to the hair shaft. Also, using Olive Oil as a serum increases the slipperiness which can prevent lice.

Prevention:

Let's first look at ways to avoid getting lice in the first place. Lice spread through hair-to-hair contact only as they do not jump, hop, or fly. The most obvious first step is to tie up long hair and teach your children not to get their heads near to children who have lice. Don't share hairbrushes, hats, etc. Also, if you have had an outbreak of lice make sure that you wash your bedding immediately in hot water and iron the bedding too. Once all of that is in place you could look at using one of more of the following on your hair to prevent infestation:

Tea Tree Oil

Rub a little tea tree oil into your hair, especially around the ears and the base of the neck. Lice don't like the smell so will stay away from hair with tea tree oil on it.

Olive Oil

After washing your hair, rub a small amount of Olive Oil into your hair to keep it nice and slippery, even if a louse does get into your hair it won't be able to lay eggs and you will avoid an infestation of nits.

Rosemary Essential Oil

Lice don't like rosemary oil, so add a few drops to your hairbrush and brush it through your hair. Interestingly, rosemary is said to combat mental tiredness, loss of motivation and memory, giving you an extra boost for your day. Other essential oils such as lavender, eucalyptus and peppermint are also just as effective.

Treatment:

If you discover lice or nits in your hair, treat it immediately with mayonnaise. This method is messy but highly effective. The mayonnaise blocks the breathing holes of the lice and smothers them. Not only will you be lice free but you will also have soft, shiny hair afterwards.

Results:

- Kills lice and nits
- Save money
- Shiny, soft hair
- No harmful chemicals

Cautions:

- Take care to wash and rinse well or greasy hair will result.
- Use shop bought mayonnaise and not a homemade one as this contains unpasteurised egg and you can run the risk of getting salmonella poisoning if you leave it in your hair too long.

NATURE'S WAY HEAD LICE TREATMENT

Ingredients: Mayonnaise

Method: Coat your hair well with room temperature mayonnaise and leave in from two to four hours.

After some time the mayonnaise gets a bit runny and will start running down your face and neck. Wrap your hair up in a plastic bag or shower cap using cotton wool around the edges to catch the runny mayonnaise.

Before washing the mayonnaise out, run a metal nit comb through your hair to remove all the nits.

Repeat daily until there are no more lice in the hair.

Repeat the treatment again in 10 days to kill any eggs that may have remained and hatched.

More head lice recipes:

There are other simple ways to get rid of lice using natural ingredients, here are some examples:

Olive Oil

Olive Oil does the same as mayonnaise but is a little easier to wash out of the hair. Castor oil does the same as Olive Oil.

Hair Straighteners or Curlers

Hot iron straightening or curling melts the nit glue and kills lice, which is very effective in getting rid of a lice problem.

Your Head Lice Treatment Experiment

Date Started_____   Date Ended_____

Recipe Used

_____

_____

_____

_____

_____

_____

Findings

_____

_____

_____

_____

_____

_____

Six month review

_____

_____

Hair Care Tips

- Brush your hair with a natural bristle brush. The natural fibres distribute the hair's natural oils from the scalp and through the hair all the way to the ends.

- Brush your scalp too. This stimulates the sebaceous gland, which in turn produces more sebum which helps build up the skins natural protective layer.

- To avoid frizzy hair don't rough dry when blow drying. Use your brush to blow dry and avoid unnecessary frizz. Also, always finish off your hair with the 'cool' button to close the cuticles and give your hair a smooth finish.

- Keep your hair hydrated and shiny by drinking lots of water.

- Wash and rinse your hair with cool water as hot water tends to dry your hair out and leave it looking dull.

- Sleep on a silk pillow case. Silk doesn't absorb moisture like cotton and is fantastic for your hair and skin.

- Exercise, sleep and diet can greatly affect your hair. Taking care of these areas will not only keep you healthy but will also ensure that you have great looking hair.

- Wet your hair before swimming so that your hair doesn't soak up the chlorinated water.

- Avoid using plastic brushes or combs as they create static electricity.

- When conditioning avoid putting oil products near the roots. Condition from about an inch away from the scalp as your roots already contain oils and don't need the extra conditioning oil.

Did you know?

- Everyone loses on average between 50 and 100 strands of hair every day. New hair grows to replace the shed hair.

- Crash dieting can trigger temporary hair loss.

ANGELA DE SOUZA

SKIN

Modern chemical filled cosmetics cause our skin to lose its natural oils and nutrients which leads to unhealthy skin and premature ageing. Not only do these chemicals affect our beauty but they are also absorbed into the blood stream and can cause all sorts of ill health. Many every day, common ingredients from your kitchen cupboards or fruit bowl can offer simple ways to achieve healthy and beautiful skin.

The most important thing is to experiment until you find what works best for you. Everyone has different skin so there cannot be one simple solution. What might work for one person might be damaging to another person. Get to know your skin type and find what works best for you.

Cleanser

Most women are oblivious to how bad facial cleansers are for them, some are even worse than soap. Chemical facial cleansers strip the skin's lipids, essential oils and anti-oxidant properties which make the face more prone to cell damage and wrinkles. The best way forward is to use natural ingredients that stimulate the skin to produce more collagen and elastin.

You might want to skip cleansing your face in the morning and leave the good bacteria on your face. This can act as a natural mild sun protection and will keep your skin better protected from the bad bacteria. Over washing your face can be just as damaging as not washing your face at all. "Many people have the concept that skin needs to be squeaky clean," explains Hema Sundaram, MD, a Washington, DC-area dermatologist and laser expert. "But that means it's been stripped of its protective barrier. We must recondition ourselves on what clean skin means, which is dewy but not tight,"

I tend to use lukewarm water just to wash sleep from my eyes in the morning. It has never felt right to wash my face twice a day, although I have not had any scientific information to back this, I just used my gut instinct that too much washing can't be good.

Nature's Way Alternatives

I have struggled with acne since my late teens and have been on various treatments, including the Dianette pill as well as Roacutane and have used the most expensive skin care products – all to no avail.

Since using Nature's Way products on my skin, I have noticed a significant change. This change was what I have desired most of my life but never managed to achieve with chemical products. You will be very surprised to hear that my skin care routine consists of lemon juice as a cleanser, mint or rose water as a toner, Olive Oil as a moisturiser and occasional exfoliating with Bicarbonate of Soda. For a treat I used a yoghurt and egg mask. It really is that simple!

Lemon juice does wonders for all skin types as well as for acne. It will kill bacteria on the surface of your skin and can cause stinging if you do have acne, but only for the first two weeks or so. In some cases it could lighten your skin and is very good for reducing acne scarring.

Lemons contain potassium and vitamin C giving your immune system a boost. They also contain Alpha Hydroxy

Acids that are a vital property for combating the causes of acne. Drinking lemon juice mixed with water is also very good for your skin.

Results:

- Healthy skin
- Save lots of money
- Natural antiseptic
- No harmful chemicals

Cautions:

- Take care not to get lemon in your eyes, it will sting a little.
- Lemon can bleach your skin but not past your natural colour.
- Using lemon or vinegar after a Bicarbonate of Soda scrub too often can cause spots.

NATURE'S WAY CLEANSER

Ingredients: Lemon Juice

Method: Squeeze a few drops of juice from a lemon and

wash your face. Rinse with warm water followed by a cold water splash for best results. It will sting on open wounds but this is not harmful.

More cleanser recipes:

There are many other simple ways to keep your skin clean using natural ingredients, here are some examples:

Olive Oil

Oil dissolves oil. Using Olive Oil not only cleanses but also nourishes your skin at the same time. Use Olive Oil to cleanse as follows:

- Rub a small amount of Olive Oil into your skin

- Begin massaging the oil into your face. This will remove all dirt and impurities. There is no need to remove makeup or wash your face beforehand.

- Remove the Olive Oil either by washing away with a warm, wet face cloth or wipe away the oil with cotton wool.

- If you use the face cloth method, hold it onto your face until it's cool then gently wipe your face. If you do this two or three times you will feel your pores releasing all the impurities leaving your skin clean and glowing.

Grapes

Grapes are a great source of OPCs which promote collagen and elastin. They are also full of natural compounds that contain antioxidant and anti-inflammatory properties which help promote blood vessel resilience for skin health. Use grapes to cleanse as follows:

- Cut a few grapes in half and gently rub them across your face for several minutes.
- Rinse with cool water

My Facial Cleanser Experiment

Date Started_____   Date Ended_____

Recipe Used

_____

_____

_____

_____

_____

_____

Findings

_____

_____

_____

_____

_____

_____

Six month review

_____

_____

Toner

Using a toner is an extra step in your skin care regime that will tighten up your pores and improve the texture of your skin. A toner can also delay natural sagging of your skin which will keep you looking younger for longer. Sadly, most chemical toners will cause harmful substances to build up in your skin which will actually damage your skin and cause premature ageing. Most toners contain alcohol, which are drying and irritating to the skin and it strips the skin of its natural protective barrier, amongst other harmful ingredients.

Using a toner will bring your skin's pH level back to normal, remove the leftover traces of dirt and make-up and will absorb the excess oil from the surface of your skin.

Nature's Way Alternatives

It's so simple that you might have overlooked this one. A splash of cool water onto your face is a great basic toner. If the water is too cold it can constrict the blood flow, and can lead to burst capillaries. Also, water that is too cold makes your face blotchy and irritated. It's best to use slightly warm water to wash and slightly cooler water to rinse as a mild toner. Of course this won't remove any traces of make-up and doesn't offer any pH balance so try using a dash of rose water or even some homemade mint water. I have also heard that apple cider vinegar does wonders as a toner. The most important thing is to experiment as everyone's skin is different and will respond differently.

Results:

- Remove traces of dirt
- Balance your skin's pH level
- Tighten your skin
- Shrink your pores
- Save lots of money
- No harmful chemicals

Cautions:

- Never apply toner to dirty skin

NATURE'S WAY TONER

Ingredients: Mint

Method: Pour hot water over fresh mint leaves or a mint

---

tea bag in a coffee cup. Leave for ten minutes. Strain and cool. Apply to your face and neck using cotton pads.

More toner recipes:

There are many other simple ways to tone your skin using natural ingredients, here are some examples:

Rose Water

Rosewater is a rich composition which enhances the skin's natural healing properties. It can be used to soothe irritations and reduce swelling and blemishes. Rosewater is an excellent daily skin toner.

- Sprits your face with rose water or use cotton pads to wipe the rose water over your face.

Cucumber and Yoghurt

- Take 1 small peeled cucumber and place it in a blender until it becomes a thick liquid paste.
- Add ½ cup plain white yoghurt
- Mix together and apply to your face and neck.
- Leave for 5-10 minutes, rinse off with lukewarm water and then rinse with cooler water to close skin pores.

Apple Cider Vinegar

Apple cider vinegar comes from fermented apples and is full of vitamins and minerals that help restore skin's pH balance. It also has antibacterial properties to fight skin infection and cleanse.

- Dilute one part apple cider vinegar in eight parts water.
- Apply to your skin and leave on from ten minutes and up to 1 hour depending on skin sensitivity.

My Facial Toner Experiment

Date Started_____   Date Ended_____

Recipe Used

_____

_____

_____

_____

_____

_____

Findings

_____

_____

_____

_____

_____

_____

Six month review

_____

_____

Moisturiser

A recent study published in the Journal of Investigative Dermatology has potentially linked the use of daily moisturizers with skin cancer. Allen Conney at Rutgers University found that skin cancer tumours increased up to 95% in high risk mice when treated with four different daily moisturizers. It is frightening to think that our daily skin care regime could be causing cancer. If you are not already discarding your shop bought beauty products and using Nature's Way, seriously consider doing so right away.

Since using Nature's Way cleansers and toners I have found that I don't need a moisturiser. Firstly, sticking to the rule of not washing my face in the morning has done wonders. All the natural goodness that my skin produces overnight is left on as a protective barrier during the day. Secondly, I find I don't need to moisturise *because* natural oils are produced as I sleep at night. Having a good cleanser and toner is sufficient to keep the natural oil production of my skin balanced. However, your skin might be different and you might feel that you need to use a moisturiser and the best thing to use is Olive Oil.

Nature's Way Alternatives

Although you can use Olive Oil as a cleanser that has

moisturising benefits, you can also use it as a moisturiser. It is filled with vitamins and natural goodness and is known to have healing properties too. Using Olive Oil doesn't cause spots and if rubbed into your skin it will actually help maintain the skin's oil balance and prevent overproduction of sebum. Using Olive Oil will also prevent water loss and restore the barriers that will renew, maintain and repair your skin.

Results:

- Healthy skin
- Removes traces of dirt
- Restores natural oil balance
- Save lots of money
- No harmful chemicals

NATURE'S WAY MOISTURISER

Ingredients: Olive Oil

Method: Rub a few drops of Olive Oil into your face and neck in the evening for added moisturising benefits.

More moisturiser recipes:

There are many other simple ways to moisturise your skin using natural ingredients, here are some examples:

Chickpea, Turmeric and Honey

Chickpea is a gentle skin exfoliator and honey moisturises. Chickpeas help skin cells produce energy to fights free-radical damage that causes wrinkles. Honey is also a natural anti-oxidant so it will help protect the skin from UV damage and aid in cell renewal. Turmeric helps to reduce pigmentation on your face and even out your skin tone. It can also greatly reduce the appearance of acne. Chickpea, turmeric and honey have enough benefits between them to warrant an entire separate book so we will leave it at that for now.

- Mix ½ teaspoon chickpea powder with a pinch of turmeric and honey.
- Blend together with milk for dry skin or Yoghurt for oily skin.
- Use your fingers to gently rub the Chickpea and Honey in a upward circling motion on your face.

Honey

Mix together 2 tablespoons of honey and 2 teaspoons of milk for an effective moisturiser.

My Facial Moisturiser Experiment

Date Started_____   Date Ended_____

Recipe Used

_____

_____

_____

_____

_____

_____

Findings

_____

_____

_____

_____

_____

_____

Six month review

_____

_____

Face Masks

There are so many weird and wonderful things that you can use to make a facial mask. My daughters and I have had loads of fun with natural masks and also had great results. Many chemical masks have frighteningly high risks so soaking your face with them is not a good idea. Most masks contain dangerous substances and block your pores. It is important to allow your skin to breathe and adding too many products can have an adverse effect.

Less is more when it comes to your skin so find a beauty regime that allows your skin to find a natural balance. Most of the time what you put into your body has more effect that what you put onto your skin. Eating healthy, exercising, sleeping well and drinking lots of water are the most important ingredients for the best looking skin.

After that comes a simple cleanse, tone and moisturise routine with natural ingredients. If necessary, use a Nature's Way mask from time to time. The best thing to help your skin get the boost it needs is a facial massage which is known to improve the circulation to your skin and will rejuvenate your face.

Here follows a simple facial massage:

Facial Massage

1. Apply a little olive oil or facial essential oil to your face.
2. Use your finger tips to massage upwards and outwards in a circular motion, starting from your chin. Start small and make the circles bigger as you move to the top of your forehead.
3. For added benefits continue your massage into your scalp as if shampooing your hair.

Nature's Way Alternatives

If you decide that you need a mask, try avocado for dry skin, green tea masks for sensitive skin, strawberry with yoghurt for oily skin and oats with lemon for acne prone skin. An egg white mask is suitable for all skin types. Egg whites are high in protein which feeds your skin and as the egg dries it tightens your skin while drawing excess oil from the pores.

Eating eggs is also great for your skin as they contain selenium, vitamins A and E, folate, riboflavin, choline and lutein. Some studies have suggested that eating eggs will smooth your skin.

Results:

- Healthier skin

- Removes fine lines

- Save lots of money

- No harmful chemicals

Cautions:

- Don't use a mask too often as it isn't necessary.

NATURE'S WAY MASKS

Ingredients: Egg White

Method: Whisk the egg whites until they get foamy. Smooth the white onto your face in an upward motion, applying liberally. Allow to dry for twenty minutes and then rinse off with warm water.

More mask recipes:

There are many other simple ways to make masks using natural ingredients, here are some examples:

Avocado (best for drier skin types)

Mash together the flesh of an avocado and apply to your face. Rinse off after ten minutes. You can also include a teaspoon of honey and a teaspoon of yoghurt to your avocado for added benefits.

Strawberry (best for oily or combination skin types)

Mix equal quantities of fresh strawberries and yoghurt. Apply to your face and rinse off after ten minutes.

Green Tea (best for sensitive skin types)

Soak a green tea bag in a quarter cup of boiling water. When cooled sufficiently, soak some cotton wool with the green tea and dab it onto your face liberally. Allow the green tea to dry naturally and don't rinse off.

Another alternative which will need washing off after ten minutes is to mix a little oats and honey into the green tea to create a face paste.

My Face Mask Experiment

Date Started_____   Date Ended_____

Recipe Used

_____

_____

_____

_____

_____

_____

Findings

_____

_____

_____

_____

_____

_____

Six month review

_____

_____

Exfoliator

Exfoliation is a good practise for removing the top layer of the skin, which consists mainly of dead skin cells, oil, sweat and dirt. As this layer builds up, it dulls your skin's appearance. Once this layer is removed, your skin will appear healthier and have a lovely natural glow to it.

Exfoliating has been around for quite some time, the Ancient Greeks exfoliated by rubbing their skin with a mixture of oils and sand. They then scraped their skin with a strigil, which is a curved metal scraper used to scrape dirt and sweat from the body before effective soaps became available.

We have moved on from that method but many modern methods can be harmful and even dangerous. Abrasive methods have long been hailed as the cure for wrinkles, acne and other skin conditions but these harsh methods actually remove your skin's natural defences. The result is not wrinkle free, acne free skin but rather damaged skin. Some exfoliators are so harsh that they can cause the face to bleed, especially ones that include sharp objects such as apricot kernels and walnut shells. These can be used for feet and elbows but definitely not for your face! Acclaimed facialists Sarah Chapman and Vaishaly Patel suggest you avoid the new breed of home microdermabrasion kits which sandblast the skin with aluminium oxide crystals. They say that these sorts of things are simply too harsh and aggressive.

A good rule of thumb is to use exfoliators that are rounded such as sand, sugar, salt, etc. If you live near the seaside I highly recommend spending some time gently rubbing the sea sand all over your body – the combination of salt and sand does wonders for your skin.

Men who shave with blade razors as opposed to electric ones don't need to exfoliate; the razor does the job quite nicely.

Nature's Way Alternatives

Ground oats is my favourite exfoliator as I always have plenty of it in my home and it does the job perfectly. Because oats are mildly rough, they are one of nature's most effective exfoliators. They soften the skin leaving it silky smooth and have been clinically shown to help heal dry, itchy skin.

Results:
- Healthier skin
- Slows the ageing process
- Save lots of money
- No harmful chemicals

Cautions:

- Don't rub too harshly or excessively.

- Avoid the delicate skin around your eyes.

- Don't exfoliate in the morning - exfoliating your face can increase sun sensitivity by up to 45% as it removes the natural oils produced while you sleep which can act as a natural mild sun protection.

- Don't use harsh exfoliators such as apricot kernel and walnut shells.

- Don't use chemical exfoliators or chemical peels as they will damage your skin.

- Don't exfoliate more than once a week – it's not necessary and can dry out or damage your skin which needs time to restore its natural oil balance.

NATURE'S WAY EXFOLIATOR

Ingredients: Oats

Method: Take 2 - 3 teaspoons of raw oats and crush them into smaller bits either by hand or in a grinder. After cleansing your face, gently rub the oats into your skin for 10 - 15 seconds. Rinse your face with warm water until

---

you no longer feel the granules of the oats. Dry your face gently with a clean soft towel and if necessary follow with a natural toner and moisturiser.

More exfoliator recipes:

Here are other simple ways to make exfoliators:

Yoghurt and Rice Powder

If you have oily skin, you can use yoghurt to exfoliate as it will remove blackheads and whiteheads.

- Mix rice powder and yoghurt together into a thick paste.
- Rub it into your skin in little circular movements.
- Leave for five minutes and rinse it off.

Olive Oil and Sugar

- 3 tablespoons of Extra Virgin Olive Oil
- ½ cup of granulated sugar
- 2 tablespoons Aloe Vera (optional)

Mix all the ingredients together and rub it into your skin in little circular movements. This is suitable for face and body exfoliation. Leave for three to five minutes and rinse it off. The sugar will remove dead skin cells and the Olive Oil and Aloe Vera will nourish your skin keeping it moisturized.

Milk and Salt

- ½ cup cold milk
- ½ tablespoon salt

Soak a cotton ball and gently dab all over your face. Allow the mixture to dry on your face for about three minutes and then dip the cotton ball in the mixture again and rub lightly in a circular motion. Rinse with warm water. The milk will remove deep pore dirt and the salt will exfoliate.

My Exfoliator Experiment

Date Started_____   Date Ended_____

Recipe Used

_____

_____

_____

_____

_____

_____

Findings

_____

_____

_____

_____

_____

_____

Six month review

_____

_____

Oils

Baby oil, along with other common household oils for massage, hair, and bath, essential oils, eucalyptus and camphor oils, are responsible for at least 3000 reported ingestion accidents to young children every year in Australia.

Toxicologist Dr Naren Gunja from NSW Poisons Information Centre at Westmead Hospital says most parents don't realise the danger. "Once the child has ingested it depending on how much they ingest then it could be too late. Over a period of time, the child can die," says Dr Gunja. "It is a gradual process that can take several days, two weeks to die."[viii]

Mineral Oils

White oil, mineral oil and more commonly known as baby oil when we buy it for our little ones, is a petroleum by-product. I don't know about you but I don't feel so good about rubbing anything from petrol all over my body, let alone my baby's body. This oil is used on its own or as a base for many other cosmetic products. It has been shown to increase the risk of cancer and is also known to trigger asthma.

This mineral oil coats the skin like cling film which inhibits its ability to breathe and absorb moisture or nutrition. Even though you might use oil to keep your skin from drying out, you will find over a period of time that it actually causes dryness and irritation and will compound the very problems you were trying to fix. When using these oils you will disrupt the skin's natural immune barrier as well as its ability to release toxins. The result is blocked pores which can lead to spots or acne and other skin disorders. It will also slow down the skin's normal functions and cell development which will cause your skin to age prematurely.

Plant Oils

Plant oils that we use in our kitchen or on our body are either heat extracted oils, expeller pressed or cold pressed oils. You would think that because it is a plant based oil that it will be safer for you than mineral oils. Sadly, even these oils can be dangerous so you need to choose wisely before eating or applying these oils to your body.

There are three methods of extracting vegetable oils from nuts, grains, beans, seeds or olives: heat extracted oils, expeller pressed oils and cold pressed oils. Cold pressed oils are the most natural oils to use. You will usually find the cold pressed oils much more expensive than heat extracted or expeller pressed oils so if you are not sure, the price will definitely be a giveaway!

Heat Extracted Oils

Extracting oil with this method is done by heating up the raw materials and possibly even adding chemicals to help extract more oil. Heat pressing increases the yielded quantity of oil which is why cold pressed oils are more expensive than heat pressed oils.

The introduction of heat and chemicals to the process of making oil degrades their flavour, nutritional value and colour. Oils are composed of long-chain fatty acids and these are damaged by heat extraction method. Little pieces break off the long-chain fatty acid when heated and are toxic to the body.

A solvent is often added to assist with the extraction. Usually a petroleum by-product like Hexane, Pentane, Heptane is used and then removed again afterwards by distillation.

Expeller Pressed Oils

Expeller pressing is a mechanical method for extracting oil from raw materials. This uses a screw or continuous press with a constantly rotating worm shaft where raw material goes in one end and is put under continuous pressure and discharged at the other end, producing oil. It is during this process that temperatures can rise up to 250°C as a result of friction. Expeller pressed oil is similar to cold pressed oil in that neither process involves the use of any chemicals. The difference between expeller pressing and the cold press method is heat. Both use presses but the cold pressed method is done in a temperature-controlled setting.

Cold Pressed Oils

Cold pressing is an ancient method and yields the best quality oil. The only two materials that will yield enough oil without requiring heat are sesame seeds and olives. These oils are the most natural form of oil and have great colour, odour and flavour. If oil has been extracted by hydraulic press but has been heated prior to pressing, it will be referred to it as pressed, not *cold* pressed so read your labels carefully. When choosing oil you need extra virgin cold pressed oil. Unrefined is always best as well as undistilled.

Nature's Way Oils

Extra virgin cold pressed oils are the only oils that you should be consuming or using on your body.

Choosing Your Oil

- **Light** - Olive Oil can become rancid from exposure to light and heat, so choose an olive oil that comes in a dark tinted glass bottle.

- **Temperature** – Buy olive oil that has been kept in cool area, away from any direct or indirect contact with heat. Cold pressed extra virgin olive oil is always best.

- **Acidity** – Extra virgin olive oil can contains up to 0.8% of free acidity. Any more than that is not extra virgin.

- **Purity** – This term can be misleading. You do **not** want pure olive oil, this means that it's a mixture of olive oils or has been purified by one of many methods that strips the oil of it nutrients. Cloudy olive oil is a good sign not a bad sign.

Sadly, to see the words "extra virgin olive oil" on the label of a bottle does not guarantee that you are getting extra virgin olive oil. You really need to know what you are looking for, the oil you are looking for is not commonly found and is not cheap.

Castor Oil

Castor Oil has many healing properties. The same properties that make it so effective in healing the body also make it an excellent choice for maintaining healthy skin and hair. For skin, castor oil not only cures acne but it also keeps the skin smooth and looking youthful. Don't bother with buying anti-ageing creams; all you need is a little castor oil rubbed around your eyes at bed time.

For hair, Castor Oil is fantastic, not only to strengthen your hair but also to encourage growth. Rubbing castor oil on your roots and scalp will regenerate new hair growth.

My Oil Experiment

Date Started_____   Date Ended_____

Recipe Used

_____

_____

_____

_____

_____

_____

Findings

_____

_____

_____

_____

_____

_____

Six month review

_____

_____

Talc

Researchers have warned that "*women should stop using talcum powder because of the risk of ovarian cancer*", reported *The Daily Telegraph. "Scientists fear particles applied to the private parts may travel to the ovaries and trigger a process of inflammation that allows cancer cells to flourish. Although previous studies have raised concerns over talc, the latest findings from the United States suggest woman who use it are 40 per cent more likely to get ovarian cancer – a much greater risk than first thought.*

Talc is made from a soft mineral called hydrous magnesium silicate, which is found throughout the world. It is crushed, dried and milled to produce powder used in cosmetic products by millions. Some experts say it has chemical similarities to asbestos, which can cause a deadly form of lung cancer." [ix]

In other research talcs have been found to lead to cognitive problems, lymphoma, breast cancer, cancer and many other issues. All in all, it's best to stay away from talc, especially with babies although talc is also found in face powders.

Nature's Way Alternatives

Corn flour is my favourite talc. I love the texture and it is super absorbent too. Corn flour mixed with bicarbonate of soda is a wonderful deodorant or underarm powder too. Other non-toxic powders that absorb moisture and keep the skin dry include bicarbonate of soda, chickpea powder, oat flour, powdered lavender buds and powdered rose petals, which can easily be found at a grocery or health shop.

Results:

- No health risks
- No harmful chemicals
- Save lots of money
- Absorbs odours
- Absorbs sweat
- Prevents nappy rash
- Prevents chafing

Cautions:

- Bicarbonate of soda can dry skin out so if you find this a problem for you, mix half corn flower and half bicarbonate of soda.
- The powdered lavender and rose petals are a bit more expensive that the flours.
- Do not inhale the powder, as this may cause breathing problems.
- Keep powders in a sealed container otherwise they

will absorb moisture and go hard.

NATURE'S WAY TALCUM POWDER

Ingredients: Corn Flour

Method: Use corn flour as you would usually use talcum powder.

More talcum powder recipes:

There are many other simple ways to make talcum powder using natural ingredients, here are some examples:

Essential Oil Powder

Mix equal portions of corn flour and bicarbonate of soda together. Add a few drops of your favourite fragrant essential oil.

Kaolin Powder

Use as a powder on its own or with other powders and essential oils. Kaolin clay is high in mineral content and lightly draws out impurities and toxins from the skin. This is particularly good for sensitive, dry or mature skin as well as for children.

Kaolin powder as a face mask ingredient assists in improving vascular and lymphatic flow. Excellent for removing impurities. Recommended for congested skin types.

My Talc Experiment

Date Started_____   Date Ended_____

Recipe Used

_____

_____

_____

_____

_____

_____

Findings

_____

_____

_____

_____

_____

_____

Six month review

_____

_____

Deodorant

Parabens are used as a preservative in most beauty products these days. Scientists have only just started looking into the dangers of parabens and there is emerging data linking parabens and cancer - especially breast cancer. One of the recent shocking discoveries is that deodorant is high in parabens and aluminium which could be one of the most significant causes of breast cancer. Chemicals can seep through your skin and get into the immediate and nearby underlying soft tissue.

Aluminium is a neurotoxin which means that it causes damage to nerves or nerve tissue. Studies have linked aluminium as a neurotoxin to Alzheimers and other neurological diseases. As stated by the FDA: *"Antiperspirants have an aluminium-based compound as their main, active ingredient, which can be any number of compounds within an established concentration and dosage form."*[x] Using aluminium on your skin is risky as it is quickly absorbed into your system and into your brain.

Even men are at risk. Many people don't realise that men can get breast cancer because you wouldn't really say that men have 'breasts'. But men do have a small amount of breast tissue behind their nipples and this is where breast cancer can develop. I have also discovered in my research that deodorants can even cause prostate cancer.

Antiperspirants are even worse – double trouble - as they stop you from sweating! Sweating is one of the ways the body cleanses itself of toxins. Antiperspirants cause the toxins in your sweat to become trapped and breast tissue is especially efficient at storing these poisons. We need to sweat; it is natural and necessary to sweat.

Nature's Way Alternatives

I used Bicarbonate of Soda as a deodorant. Simply use it as you would a talcum powder but of course talcum powder is a big 'no no'. It's simple and highly effective. Armpit odour is caused by bacteria present on the skin's surface. Bicarbonate of Soda has strong antibacterial properties and so is the simplest alternative for chemical deodorants.

Results:
- No harmful chemicals
- Clean bacteria free armpits
- No cancer risks
- Save money
- Natural toxin excretion
- No white marks on clothes

Cautions:

- Slight burning or a rash might occur at first as your underarms detox but this does pass.

NATURE'S WAY DEODORANT

Ingredients: Bicarbonate of Soda

Method: Apply under your arms with a powder puff or a Kabuki brush. You can also add some corn flour to your Bicarbonate of Soda to make it a little gentler to apply.

More deodorant recipes:

There are many recipes available for homemade deodorants using natural ingredients, here are some:

Essential Oil and Bicarbonate of Soda

- 1/4 cup Corn Flour
- 1/4 cup Bicarbonate of Soda
- 10 drops of Essential Oil
- 2 Tablespoons Shea Butter

Mix all ingredients together very well and into a deodorant stick.

Lemon

- Fresh Lemon

Rub half a lemon under your arms once or twice a day to kill bacteria and give you a nice fresh smelling arm pit.

Coconut Oil

- 1/4 cup Corn Flour
- 1/4 cup Bicarbonate of Soda
- 10 drops of Essential Oil
- 2 Tablespoons Coconut Oil

Mix all ingredients together well to get a creamy lotion. To create a solid stick put your mixture in the fridge. Coconut oil solidifies below 24.5°C. Rub on like an ordinary deodorant.

My Deodorant Experiment

Date Started_____   Date Ended_____

Recipe Used

_____

_____

_____

_____

_____

_____

Findings

_____

_____

_____

_____

_____

_____

Six month review

_____

_____

Body Wash

'Women who use shower gels and soaps in intimate areas are putting themselves at higher risk of developing sexually transmitted infections, experts have warned.

Researchers at the University of California, Los Angeles, say that soaps and lubricants can damage sensitive tissues and raise a woman's chance of becoming infected with herpes, chlamydia and HIV.

Study leader Joelle Brown said there is 'mounting evidence' that using these products internally can increase the risk of bacterial vaginosis – a condition that occurs when the bacterial balance becomes disrupted - and sexually transmitted infections."

Daily Mail, Online Article 2296929

Doctors do not recommend that women wash themselves internally at all because it can alter the balance of bacteria. Soap and shower gel is a definite no no for our girly bits but what about the rest of our body? Does washing the rest of our body alter the skins natural bacteria balance too? How safe is it to use a cocktail of chemicals to cleanse ourselves? Do you really know how much of what you wash yourself with is absorbed into your blood stream? Does washing with regular soaps or gels leave your skin feeling dry, itchy or oily? I am not going to tell you how harmful these things are, just see for yourself when you next wash and decide if your current method is working for you.

Skin and pH Balance

Skin is the largest organ of the body. It regulates body temperature, protects from environmental elements and fights off germs. But skin's power relies on something we can't even see. The acid mantle is a thin, viscous fluid that protects our skin. It consists of two fluids: sweat and sebum. Sweat glands produce a salty, watery solution that mixes with sebum, an oily secretion produced by sebaceous glands near hair follicles. The acid mantle maintains a pH between 4.0 and 5.5, a range that allows it to help skin stay healthy. The acid mantle helps our skin in a number of ways. It acts as an antioxidant, protecting underlying skin from damage. It helps repel water so skin layers are not damaged, and it inhibits bacterial growth. It also maintains the hardness of protein. Outer skin is made of a protein called Keratin that needs to have an acidic balance to stay strong, so the acid mantle helps stave off alkaline that could break up the protein and cause problems like acne and skin allergies.

Since the acid mantle plays such a key role in how our skin functions, it is necessary to protect it. Any disruption to the acid mantle will interfere with the protective shield of skin cells that surrounds the epidermis. Cells can be dislodged from each other, causing dryness, irritation, roughness and flaking. When cells break apart, skin is left defenceless. Also, as cells pull away, the remaining breaks leave skin exposed to bacteria. Usually bacteria has trouble penetrating the skin when pH is normal, because the acid mantle creates an unfavourable environment. If pH rises, the natural prevention of infection is compromised, making it easier for bacteria to penetrate under the skin, causing numerous skin problems.

It seems simple enough: Protect the acid mantle and regulate pH level to maintain healthy skin. However, it's a lot more difficult than that, especially when you consider the fact that almost everything we face in our day to day life can interfere with the acid mantle. Sunlight, diet, excessive sweating and even applying skincare products can disrupt the harmony of skin pH.

Protecting Skin pH

When it comes to skin treatment, the biggest mistake people make is washing skin with harsh soaps that are high in alkaline. As they strip off the acid mantle, these soaps debilitate natural defences and extract fats that actually help protect skin. Bacteria is free to attack and can cause infection. It's better to use a cleanser that contains more acidic or neutral elements, such as alpha hydroxyl or beta hydroxy. These will keep skin cells tightly locked together, maintaining skin's healthy glow.[xi]

Nature's Way Alternatives

For an easy and lightly scented body wash use castile

soap and essential oils. Castile soap was originally a name used for olive oil based soap made in a style similar to that originating in the Castile region of Spain. However, today castile soap refers to any soap made from mostly vegetable oils.

Results:

- No harmful chemicals
- No drying effects
- No cancer risks
- Save money

Cautions:

- When buying castile soap check that it is 100% natural vegetable oil as some may contain other ingredients.

NATURE'S WAY BODY WASH

Ingredients: Castile soap, essential oil

Method: Shred one bar castile soap using the vegetable grater and heat up in 6 cups of water until soap is fully

---

melted. When cooled, stir in 10 drops essential oil of your choice and pour into containers.

More body wash recipes:

There are many recipes available for homemade body wash using natural ingredients, here are some:

Herbal Body Wash

- 1/4 Aloe Vera gel
- 1 1/2 cups liquid castile soap
- 40 drops of Essential Oil
- 7 drops coriander Essential Oil
- 7 drops lavender Essential Oil

Mix all ingredients together very well and pour into a container.

Moisturising Body Wash

- 2 cups liquid castile soap
- 1/2 cup coconut oil
- 1/2 cup honey
- 10 drops Essential Oil

Mix all ingredients together very well and pour into a container.

Using castile soap as a base you can experiment with all sorts of natural ingredients to make a body wash that suits you and your family.   You can also use the body wash recipe as a shampoo.

My Body Wash Experiment

Date Started_____   Date Ended_____

Recipe Used

_____

_____

_____

_____

_____

_____

Findings

_____

_____

_____

_____

_____

_____

Six month review

_____

_____

MAKE UP

Lip Stick

Lipstick is usually made up of a wax mixed with oil such as mineral, castor oil or lanolin along with pigments and additives for colour and fragrance. As mentioned in the section on oils, mineral oil can clog the pores which will cause all sorts of problems. Castor oil is fantastic so a lipstick using this oil is great but lanolin, oil from lambs' wool, is a common allergen. Lipsticks can also contain ingredients such as beetles and fish scales. The Campaign for Safe Cosmetics tested thirty three lipsticks for lead, from Burt's Bees Lip Shimmer to L'Oreal Colour Riche. They found that 61% of the lipsticks tested contained a detectable amount of the contaminant. In fact, several lipsticks exceeded the Food and Drug Administration's lead limit for sweets. So why do they insist on using lead? Lead makes lipstick stay on your lips longer.

All unnatural ingredients contain a health risk and you never really know what is in your lipstick, do you? Especially the cheap ones that come from places where there is limited or no testing done. There is no reason to take a risk with something that you put on your mouth, take care to either find a lipstick that you are certain contains only natural ingredients or take a few minutes to make your own.

Nature's Way Alternatives

I use Castor Oil or Olive Oil to add a natural shine to my lips in place of a lip gloss or lip stick. Castor Oil is well known for its antibacterial, moisturising and anti-aging properties. Both oils will not only moisturise your lips but they will also feed your lips with nourishing nutrients. Using petroleum jelly for your lips suffocates your lips and offers no nutritional value. The name says it all, it comes from petrol. There are many other alternatives to lipstick as well as fantastic homemade lipsticks which look just as good as shop bought products.

Results:

- No harmful chemicals
- Anti-aging
- Natural shine
- No cancer risks
- Save money

NATURE'S WAY LIPSTICK

Ingredients: Castor Oil

Method: Smooth onto your lips with your fingers or a small lip brush as a subtle lip-gloss in place of lip-gloss or lipstick.

More lipstick recipes:

There are many recipes available for homemade lipsticks using natural ingredients, here are some:

Beeswax Lipstick

- 1 tablespoon Beeswax
- 1 tablespoon Shea Butter
- 1 tablespoon Coconut Oil
- 1 teaspoon Coco Powder or natural food colouring

Melt the first three ingredients together over a bowl of boiling water. Add cocoa or colouring and mix very well. Pour into an old washed out lipstick container or buy lip balm tins from Amazon or somewhere similar.

Cranberry Lipstick

- 1 tablespoon Shea Butter
- 1 tablespoon Castor Oil
- 10 fresh cranberries

Gently melt the ingredients together. Stir well and mash the berries. Let the mixture stand for a few minutes then strain the mixture through a fine sieve to remove all the pieces of cranberry. Pour into a lip balm container for a shiny lipstick.

My Lipstick Experiment

Date Started_____   Date Ended_____

Recipe Used

_____

_____

_____

_____

_____

_____

Findings

_____

_____

_____

_____

_____

_____

Six month review

_____

_____

Mascara

Mascara has been used as far back as the ancient Egyptian era. Dating from around 3400-30 B.C., Egyptians used bone and ivory to apply their mascara. The very first recorded mascara was a blend of kohl with crocodile dung, water and honey. The Egyptians produced mascaras in the form of pressed cakes and it wasn't until the sixties that mascara applicator brushes were introduced. Even with questionable ingredients, the lure of long, sexy eye lashes has always been found beautiful and irresistible.

Like all other chemical beauty products, mascara carries risks. Methylparaben, aluminum powder, ceteareth-20, butylparaben, or benzyl alcohol are often found in mascaras and some of these ingredients have been known to cause cancer in mice. Not all mascaras will be that dangerous but just the thought of putting those nasty chemicals that close to my eyes does make me worry a little.

Other disadvantages are that chemical mascaras can be drying to eyelashes. Waterproof mascaras are particularly harmful as they contain a chemical called dimethicone copolyol that glues the mascara to your lashes. Beauty experts say they should not be used daily but rather for infrequent special occasions.

Did you know you are supposed to throw your mascara away every three to six months to prevent bacteria building up in your mascara?

Nature's Way Alternatives

I use Castor Oil. You can use an old mascara applicator you've sterilised to apply or simply use your finger tip. Castor Oil keeps them moist and will promote growth resulting in thicker and longer eye lashes. There is no risk to your eyes except that Castor Oil is sticky so if you wear contact lenses apply the Castor Oil after putting your contact lenses in. Another great plus is that using Castor Oil will also cure eye styes and keep your eyes healthy. Rub or dab Castor Oil onto the infected area to treat styes. Also, rub some around your eye too before you go to bed - you will eliminate fine lines around your eyes.

Results:
- No harmful chemicals
- Anti-aging
- Thicker, longer lashes and brows
- No cancer risks
- Save money

Cautions:

- Don't apply Castor Oil anywhere near your eyes before putting contact lenses into your eyes.

- Rinse off Castor Oil from around your eyes in the morning if necessary to avoid having a sticky look and feel all day.

NATURE'S WAY MASCARA

Ingredients: Castor Oil

Method: Smooth onto your eye lashes or eye brows with your fingers, cotton bud or a sterilised applicator brush.

More mascara recipes:

There are many recipes available for homemade mascaras using natural ingredients, here are some:

Conditioning Mascara

Mix these ingredients together and apply.

- 1 tablespoon Castor Oil
- 1 tablespoon Aloe Vera Gel

- 2 tablespoons Vitamin E Oil

Charcoal Mascara

Mix food grade charcoal with your favourite oil or aloe.

- 1 activated charcoal capsule
- 4 tablespoons Castor Oil, Olive Oil, Coconut Oil or Aloe Vera Gel.

My Mascara Experiment

Date Started_____   Date Ended_____

Recipe Used

_____

_____

_____

_____

_____

_____

Findings

_____

_____

_____

_____

_____

_____

Six month review

_____

_____

Foundation

We have all seen the women who walk around looking a bit like circus clowns. Too much makeup is never a good thing and wearing too much foundation can make you look older than you are and will actually highlight spots or flaws in your skin. The best sort of foundation is one that looks as natural as possible and what better foundation than one that *is* actually natural. The following table shows the health concerns based on commonly used liquid foundation.

Health concerns of ingredients

	low	moderate	high
Overall Hazard			
Cancer			
Developmental & reproductive toxicity			
Allergies & immunotoxicity			
Use restrictions			

Other HIGH concerns: Neurotoxicity, Endocrine disruption, Persistence and bioaccumulation, Organ system toxicity (non-reproductive), Miscellaneous, Multiple, additive exposure sources, Irritation (skin, eyes, or lungs), Contamination concerns, Occupational hazards

Other LOW concerns: Ecotoxicology, Data gaps, Enhanced skin absorption

Nature's Way Alternatives

I use a combination of corn flour, cocoa, nutmeg and cinnamon for a powder foundation. Cinnamon adds a lovely glow, cocoa ads depth and of course darkness and nutmeg adds a sun kissed tone. Finely ground oats is another fantastic alternative to corn flour as it nourishes the skin with plant protein.

Results:
- No harmful chemicals
- Anti-aging
- Nourishes skin
- No cancer risks
- Save money

Cautions:
- Don't use too much foundation as you will look really unnatural.
- Ensure that you have mixed the correct colour to suit your skin.
- Don't neglect sun protection when staying in the sun for long periods of time but keep in mind that you cannot add powder foundation over sun

block as it might dissolve into the sun block and leave your face looking blotchy.

NATURE'S WAY FOUNDATION

Ingredients: Corn flour, Cocoa, Nutmeg and Cinnamon

Method: Use 1 tablespoon of corn flour as a base and slowly mix in the cocoa to get the correct shade of brown for your skin. Add cinnamon and nutmeg to get the right tone for your skin and when satisfied apply with a kabuki brush.

More foundation recipes:

There are many recipes available for homemade foundations using natural ingredients, here is one:

Bronzing Powder

Mix these ingredients together and apply.

- 2 teaspoons corn flour or finely ground oats
- 1 tablespoon of cinnamon

My Foundation Experiment

Date Started_____   Date Ended_____

Recipe Used

_____

_____

_____

_____

_____

_____

Findings

_____

_____

_____

_____

_____

_____

Six month review

_____

_____

Blusher

As with all unnatural or chemical cosmetics, your blusher could contain ingredients that are harmful to you. Parabens, fragrance, dyes and preservatives are added and used to increase the shelf life of our cosmetics. These chemicals can be found in many cosmetics, including your blusher. Blusher recipes vary but most conventional recipes also tend to contain talc. Creating your own blusher is cheap and easy so why take the chance?

Nature's Way Alternatives

Beetroot powder or arrowroot powder is all you need for blusher but to get the perfect colour you can try a few different recipes using cinnamon or cocoa powder.

Results:

- Quick and easy
- No harmful chemicals
- Healthy, natural glow
- Save money

Cautions:

- Don't overdo the reds as you will look unnatural.

NATURE'S WAY BLUSHER

Ingredients: Arrowroot Powder, Hibiscus Powder, Cocoa

Method: Use 1 teaspoon of arrowroot powder as the base and then mix in the hibiscus powder and cocoa until you get the perfect colour. Cinnamon can also be used for a little depth and glow with or in place of cocoa. Apply with a kabuki brush.

More blusher recipes:

Here are some recipes for homemade blushers:

Beetroot and Strawberry Blusher
- 1/4 cup strawberries
- 1/4 cup beetroot
- 1/2 teaspoon olive oil
- 1/2 teaspoon honey (optional)

Blend strawberries and beetroot together.
Strain through a sieve to remove solids.

Mix in the olive oil and honey to create a natural blush cream.

Rub it into your cheeks or onto your lips for a soft, glowing look.

Beetroot Blusher

Cut fresh beetroot in half, rub your finger on and apply fresh juice. It also works very well as a lip stain. Don't use too much on your cheeks though or you might end up looking like a clown! Alternatively, buy beetroot powder and apply it with your usual blusher brush.

My Blusher Experiment

Date Started_____   Date Ended_____

Recipe Used

_____

_____

_____

_____

_____

_____

Findings

_____

_____

_____

_____

_____

_____

Six month review

_____

_____

DO NOT WORRY

Your body is designed to self heal. Every single cell in our body can repair itself if our immune system is functioning well. Even damaged hair and spotty skin should be able to heal automatically. Our body is an amazing and intricate design that should function absolutely perfectly. Sadly this is not the case for most people as we neglect our bodies and damage its natural ability to repair itself. We poison our system with chemicals and we poison our mind with worry. Yes, worry and a healthy body is connected.

Research by Dr Bruce Lipton PhD suggests that '95% of illness is caused by stress'. It has also been proven that stress can cause or worsen acne. A study was conducted in 2002 by the Stanford University School of Medicine involving 22 students suffering from acne. Their findings indicated that "Subjects who had the greatest increases in stress during examination periods also had the greatest exacerbation in acne severity." Brittle, peeling nails also are a common side effect of stress. Hair loss or damage can also be caused by stress. The bottom line is that most dysfunction in our body can be traced back to one single cause – stress.

Removing every chemical from your health and beauty routine and replacing it with a Nature's Way alternative is definitely a good thing to do. But even doing this might not give you the results you desire. You see, working on the outside of our body is only one aspect of Nature's Way. Other factors are at work in our body and these factors hugely affect our health too. If 95% of illness is caused by stress then it stands to reason that 95% of our hair, teeth, nails and skin problems are caused by stress too. The key to a beautiful you could be as simple as not worrying! Worry is the most useless emotion that has no benefits, only harmful side effects.

What is worry?

To worry is to give way to anxiety or concern, to allow your mind to dwell on difficulty or troubles. Stress is the result of worry. When you worry about something it adds a weight onto your mind which has physical consequences.

How does it work?

Stress causes your body to react. Your body perceives a threat and instantly protects itself by going in to 'fight or flight' mode. This is a good thing that protects your body from danger. When you are stressed, your sympathetic nervous system signals the adrenal glands to release adrenaline and cortisol. This causes your blood flow to change and your heart to beat faster. Your body stops focusing on digestion and your immune systems stops healing your body. All this happens so that your body can give all its energy and blood flow to your muscles so that you can run away from or fight the threat. Once the stress passes, your system will return to normal. Most people's stress responses are activated often and for prolonged periods of time. This means that the body doesn't always have a chance to return to normal which as you can imagine is very dangerous. Stress is known to cause all sorts of medical conditions from a stiff neck or headache to cancer. It is also the cause of bad hair, teeth and nails.

Stress stops our body from performing its natural healing activities because it is focusing on surviving the 'threat'.

Steps to restore you balance

1. Relax

To keep your body healthy you need to activate the body's relaxation response after a fight or flight episode. Use a breathing technique that involves exhaling longer than inhaling. Count to 4 while inhaling and breathe out until a count of 5. Do this several times until your heart rate returns to normal.

2. Think Differently

Worry begins in your mind. The quickest and easiest way to stop worrying is to change the way you think about things. Simply consider that it's not as bad as it seems or change your perspective. A fresh perspective always helps!

3. Laugh

Laughter has been scientifically proven to produce endorphins which are your 'happy' hormones. Worry cannot exist where there is joy. Circumstances might not change to eliminate your worry but you can laugh rather than cry by choice most of the time. Find a funny movie, hang out with people that make you laugh or just laugh it off. You cannot change anything at all by worrying but you can change a lot by laughing.

4. Exercise

The quickest way to deal with worry is to walk it off. However, a period of intense exercise does wonders not only for your endorphin levels but also for your stress levels. If you don't have the opportunity to do some intense exercise then at least find a way to go for a brisk walk before you return to the situation that is causing worry.

So all in all, no matter how much you try and beautify yourself on the outside, you can become instantly more beautiful far quicker by simply not worrying about things anymore.

ANGELA DE SOUZA

ABOUT THE AUTHOR

Angela De Souza is the mother of four beautiful children, speaker, author, business woman and song writer. Born in Crawley, England, she spent all of her childhood in South Africa and now lives in Cheltenham with her Brazilian husband, Eric. Together, Eric and Angela are Senior Pastors of D7 Church.

Angela has a passion to see women reach their full potential. She has published many books which cover the issues keeping today's women from being free and also writes a Blog. The King's Daughters Conference is an annual UK women's conference where she continues to explore the theme of discovering the woman you were born to be.

www.kingsdaughters.co.uk
www.kingsdaughtersconference.co.uk

Other Books *by* Angela

LOVING LIFE SERIES

Hope's Journey

"There was a time when all I wanted was to die but now that I have tasted life I really don't want to die until I have truly lived!" Hope's Journey is a heart wrenching account of Angela's struggle with depression & suicide.

Hope's Journey STUDY GUIDE

We all need HOPE. Hope's Journey STUDY GUIDE is about working together to find the hope that we have lost - a practical study to help you find a healthier mental, emotional and physical life for self-study or group studies.

Secure on the Rock

Every little girl wants to know that their daddy thinks they are beautiful! As we grow older that doesn't change we still longs to hear the words, "You are beautiful". But what if your daddy didn't call you beautiful but hurt you and did things he shouldn't?

Secure on the Rock STUDY GUIDE

We have all been through "stuff" that has robbed us of our

security - it's time to take back what is rightfully ours. Secure on the Rock STUDY GUIDE is about finding security together ideal for self-study or small group studies.

Passion & Purity

"God made us girls for extravagant, wild, imaginative, adventurous, fantastic loving!" Angela openly shares of how her search for passion ended up in adultery and how she managed to find a way back to purity.

Passion & Purity STUDY GUIDE

Is your marriage lacking 'spark'? Are you good friends but not passionate lovers? Get that spark back and live as God intended you to live - with extravagant, wild, imaginative, adventurous, fantastic loving!

LIVING LIFE SERIES

Free

Living life the way it was meant to be. There has to be more to life than this! What am I here for? What is my purpose? Who am I really? I have to find myself! Am I good enough? Who am I? "*Free*" explores all these nagging questions.

Abundant Life

Living Life to the Full

Why does the Bible say that we can have life abundantly and yet so many people are still struggling? Why does the Bible say that we don't have to worry about money and yet most people still worry? How do we live the life that it Jesus wants us to live in this day and age? ABUNDANT LIFE highlights the valuable and timeless principles that lead to a life more abundantly.

He Restores My Soul

Do you ever feel like you are stuck on a treadmill that is set too fast and you cannot find the stop button? Modern living can often feel just like that at times. Stress, heart attacks, family breakdown and so much more is the result of the way we live our life these days. Press the pause button, take a deep breath, and uncover a much better way to live.

Emotional Gravity

What Goes Up Must Come Down

Do you feel a constant pull in your life but cannot explain what it is? It is gravity on your physical body but there is also emotional gravity pulling on your soul! Life is constantly in motion. Life never stands still and will always involved change. The sooner you accept this reality the sooner you will be able to lead a life without too many disappointments.

BEING SERIES

Being a Woman

"What is the true meaning of being a woman?" The heart of a woman screams to be free to love extravagantly and to live intentionally. A refreshing read with lively discussion from six women - it's NOT at all what you might think.

Being a Wife

Being a Wife is a follow on from Being a Woman where we go into the Biblical role of the wife in depth. An exciting adventure for wives of all ages, shapes, sizes and colours.

Being a Friend

Being a Friend is a part of the Being series and takes a look at how to be a great friend. Using Biblical keys, discover how to have better friendships. Complete with study guide and real discussion with a group of every day ordinary friends.

Being a Mother

Being a Mother is a valuable part of the Being series and takes a look at how to raise our children the Biblical way. In a time where parenting seems more challenging than ever before, Being a Mother offers practical information that can be used in small group study as well as individually.

Being a Lover

Being a Lover is a part of the Being series where we look at the honest and practical truth about sex. God made sex for pleasure yet most women struggle to be free in this area. A must read for women with great benefits for men too.

Being a Woman in Business

Being a Woman in Business is a fantastic addition to the Being family where we explore dynamic business principles that can be applied no matter what your gender but we will also explore how we can become successful business *women*.

Being a Woman in Ministry

Being a Women in Ministry is an honest look at life in Christian ministry. Written by a collection of women in ministry from around the world, it's a refreshing read on the many up, downs, challenges and joys of being a woman in ministry.

FICTION

Christian and Arabella

A love stronger than anything imaginable.

Imagine Catherine Cookson writing a story set in the year 2012. This would best describe Christian and Arabella. They were from two different worlds. Christian would do anything to win Arabella's heart but most of his attempts were intercepted by the cruel Randy and life itself. Arabella seemed on a downward spiral and life for her was filled with one heart ache after another. Christian never lost hope and never stopped loving her to the point that it would cost him everything. If ever there was a tale of true romance and the power of one man's love, this is it.

Astonishing and enchanting, Christian and Arabella kept intact all the details of a modern tale of passion. Sumptuously captivating, Christian and Arabella are the most unlikely match. He devotes his life to protecting her. She devotes her time to throwing her life away. He will not rest until he wins her heart and helps to restore the woman he once met, the woman he knows still exists beneath the dark exterior of Arabella.

The most romantic story ever written. A Romeo and Juliet story with a happy ending.

MONEY MATTERS

Are you tired of trying to get through each month, living only to make ends meet? Have you read all the books that promise 'seven steps to financial freedom' but lead you nowhere? Or are you someone who has plenty of money but can't find any satisfaction in life?

Money Matters has powerful, yet easy to understand principles that will radically revolutionise your view of money. Money Matters is a set of three books that will completely revolutionise your finances. Starting with simple truths to lead you to financial freedom, followed by a devotional that will assist you in renewing your mind in the area of finances and finally a workbook that offers very practical guidelines along with spreadsheets and tools for calculating your budget.

Money Matters - *Simple Truths Leading to Financial Freedom*

Money Matters Devotional - *Renewing the Mind in the Area of Finances*

Money Matters Workbook - *Sort Out Your Money One Step at a Time*

OTHER

Esther or Delilah

An honest look at how women use their beauty to seduce men! Whether you like it or not you are using your beauty for something, but are you using it to empower a man or are you using it in a way that leaves him powerless?

Nature's Way

You have the right to know that the government doesn't review the safety of products before they're sold. You have the right to practical solutions to protect yourself and your family from everyday exposures to the chemicals that modern health and beauty products contain. Exercise your rights today and begin taking care of yourself NATURE'S WAY.

Family Favourites

A collection of our family's favourite recipes. Our family

consists of British, American, Brazilian, Portuguese and South African which means that we have loads of lovely food to choose from. Our family favourites are recipes that I, Angela De Souza, grew up with from my mother, Rosalind Pattyn and recipes that Eric grew up with recipes from his mum Sueli De Souza. To my wonderful four children, take this recipe book and add your own favourites and pass this book on to your children on their wedding day. *Love Mommy xxx*

LOVING LEADERSHIP SERIES

The Tale of a Church Planter

The ups, downs, frustrations, joys and everything in-between on the roller coaster ride of church planting. I can honestly say that no recipe or formula for church building exists - God does not work in this way! D7 Church is proof of this. Not because we didn't try, we did try just about everything. It was only when we gave up and said so to God that we began to have breakthrough.

[i] www.mercola.com, Aspartame is, by Far, the Most Dangerous Substance on the Market that is Added To Foods
[ii] Augenstein WL, Spoerke DG, Kulig KW, *et al.* (November 1991). "Fluoride ingestion in children: a review of 87 cases"
[iii] Nochimson G. (2008). Toxicity, Fluoride. eMedicine. Retrieved 2008-12-28.
[iv] www.metro.co.uk/news/474348-mouthwash-can-raise-cancer-risk
[v] www.ewg.org/release/children-exposed-daily-personal-care-products-chemicals-not-found-safe-kids
[vi] www.ewg.org/news/safe-not-sorry-hair-case-nontoxic-shampoos-conditioners-and-colors
[vii] "Head-lice Lotion Poses Health Risk to Children", *The London Times*, October 5, 1997, p.3.
[viii] http://au.news.yahoo.com/today-tonight/consumer/article/-/5035273/dangers-baby-oil/
[ix] By Alastair Jamieson, 27 Sep 2008, www.telegraph.co.uk
[x] Rados, Carol. "Antiperspirant Awareness: It's Mostly No Sweat." FDA Consumer Magazine. July-Aug. 2005. US Food and Drug Adminitration. 4 Jan. 2008 http://www.fda.gov/fdac/features/2005/405_sweat.html.
[xi] www.healthyskinportal.com/articles/understanding-skin-ph-levels/260/

www.ingramcontent.com/pod-product-compliance
Lightning Source LLC
Chambersburg PA
CBHW072247310526
45795CB00011B/287